Go For It...
TAKE WHAT
YOU NEED....!

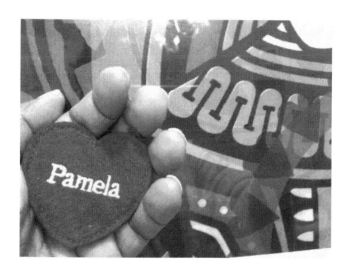

By
Pamela Rene' Slater

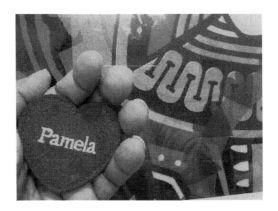

For permission requests, write to the Permissions Coordinator at the email address below.

pslater@comcast.net
SimplyAHelpmate_PRSlater@Outlook.net
goodlife@simply-a-helpmate.com
C:862.823.6029 / P:732.784.8417

Edited by the Readers...please drop me a line if you notice something...! (~_~)

ACKNOWLEDGMENTS

This book is dedicated to so many that I would have to do a separate one just to acknowledge and thank you all.

Thank you to all my favorite brothers, sisters, nieces, nephews, cousins, uncles, aunts, friends, teachers, mentors and pets!

Thank you to every person who has touched my life in so many ways with encouraging words, prayers, mentoring and motivating conversations.

Thank you to Phyllis Cunningham, Linda Price, Beloved Reese and Dr. Stephanie D. Burroughs who gently nudged me in the way that I did them while they wrote their own books.

Wishing you a great life!

Hugs!

Pam

INTRODUCTION

There is a quiet and still place that I go when I need to create balance and peace in my soul. This shift is a place where I meet my spiritual mentor who I choose to call God.

He/She/ It is called many names by others.

It really does not matter the name or not; as the important thing is the feeling of total bliss that happens when I go to this place of stillness which is a combination of prayer and meditation, a balance of all things required for my healthy mind and body. A place where spirit flows in words, sounds, images and thoughts.

When I first started, I thought sitting in stillness would help me to organize my thoughts to give my prayer and meditation practice an outlet to discover more truths about myself. At some point I started journaling.

This book is some of my experiences with the flow of that communication ending with statements that I focus on to encourage myself.

My hope is that you will...

Go For It & "Take What You Need!"

Wishing you a good life!

Pamela

TABLE OF CONTENTS

Honestly, I don't really have one but if you open this book at random what is needed will find you.

Instead, below are interests that are close to my heart.

A percentage of all sales will be gifted to them.

First Baptist Church of Linden, N.J Scholarship Guild - http://www.firstbaptistchurchoflinden.org/

Morning Star Community Christian Center of Linden, N.J. Scholarship Guild - http://morningstarccc.org/

Community Food Bank of New Jersey - http://www.cfbnj.org/

Elizabeth Coalition to House the Homeless - http://theelizabethcoalition.org/

Set Her Free – http://setherfree.org/

Someone's Daughter Organization - http://www.someonesdaughter.org/

KRYSTAL

Go For It...
TAKE WHAT
YOU NEED....!

Hugs

Pam

IN THE BEGINNIG....

In the beginning what I wrote in my journal made absolutely no sense. I wrote about who I needed to call that day, my chipped nail polish and the need for a mani-pedi as well as other nonsense.

But I kept at it whenever the nudging of a thought moved me to pen and paper in one of my note books. On one of these mornings I felt this weird shift happen in my thought, body and heart. It was an unusual feeling to my senses but not uncomfortable. I felt rather raw and exposed as the sensation began to open me up. I began to feel light, fluid; connected to a different energy and wrote the following:

Silence

It sounds like peace

It sounds like healing

It sounds like love

It sounds like pain

It sounds like goals

It sounds like tears

It sounds like manifestation

It sounds like prosperity

It sounds like the rhythm of breath bouncing to the beat of God Almighty!

Shalom

Go For It: In my silence I connect with the heartbeat of God who loves and guides me every day.

The next time my rambling thoughts started with...

Good morning.

The continued rise in colonialism perpetuates a society of moral-less humans destroying the earth. Pizza is not good dough. Man do my feet hurt.

Then I felt that same shift just like the day before and I wrote.

I'm a cool breeze on a hot sweltering day. There is a skip boopity bump to my stride. I'm a cool cat. I got it like that. My stroke is fluid. I sing when I speak with fluidity causing fine as wine to strip bare their most prized possessions bending knees when I pass.

Trees bow their bark and leaves quiver in ecstasy when I walk under them for shade. I walk to the boopity bop. My God given right to walk and flow.

So now I'm thinking this is interesting and that I must have read it somewhere!

However, soon I discover that these were just practice exercises to help me get in touch with my own thoughts until I learned to listen intuitively to God.

They were preparation and drills to center my mind, body and spirit.

This still continues at random to this day with thoughts like......Well, well, well good morning. How did I sleep last night? What age is retirement?"

And next comes the shift...

MAN IS THE SUM

Man is the sum of all of his experiences. This includes past and present journeys as well as many life times. Heaven is real and so is reincarnation.

Blasphemy! Did I just write that man can live many times? Could it be true that man can live and does live many lives? Do we choose to forget? Forgetting is convenient and makes us less accountable. Except now is the time.

So, I kept at my rambling writing.

Now is the time where consciousness is high, and those excuses are lies. We do know, and we need to recognize that we have a purpose. This requires change. This change requires dedication to our Maker. This change requires commitment. This change requires faith to complete our purpose. This change requires manifesting good. This change requires the action of sowing.

This change is global and until we own this change. Man will suffer the consequence for ignoring what has been taught in the past, present and future for it is written. Shalom

Oh goodness what does this mean? I thought I was just going to write a light and breezy book on my discovery of self with poems, some pretty photos and drawings.

Oh well...see what you think!

"Please Take What You Need!"

Go For It: My past, present and future steps are ordered by a Father who is concerned about my growth

NOW IS THE TIME

Now is the time for all to come to the realization that developing purpose is solely up to them.

No one will pressure you.

Now one will even push you. Unless you ask for it aware or unaware!

For asking or not is receiving exactly what you are entitled to. Entitlement comes with responsibility. But remember you asked for it.

Therefore, why complain when the thing you asked for appears in your life.

Instead embrace the opportunity to have or meet a new challenge. Each new challenge is filled with excitement and/or fear depending on how you look at it and who you trust.

Trusting in self is good but not nearly enough to succeed.

Trust needs to come from a place so deeply rooted inside your inner most being. This kind of trust is a knowing feeling. It's a feeling that warms you in that fuzzy tingling sort of way. It makes your eyes sparkle, your soul sing and your steps light.

For now, your steps are ordered by a higher connection that is available to help you.

Embrace this help for this too is part of your birth right. It will help you succeed because you asked for it!

Go For It: I embrace help from my Higher Power to receive everything that I am entitle to by birth right. I trust this guidance will help me succeed in fulfilling my purpose.

THE EYE OF GOD

Let's consider seeing truth in all things.

Do we really believe that only one religion is going to heaven?

Do we really believe that only one faith has favor with the Infinite?

Now I was raised Christian and for me there is something about Jesus that moves the depth of my soul.

However, I can see that same energy that I have for Jesus, God and the Holy Spirit manifesting goodness in believers of Buddha, Krishna, Mohammed, and Jehovah for all humans.

For aren't we all a type of Jesus misunderstood?

A misunderstanding regarding who can call him Father?

When you really think about it, any of us who can't call God Father are really missing the mark because the eye of God is cellular in all things.

We are all a living part of Him which makes us all part of the same life force no matter what you choose to call it.

Go For It: I am an individual part of the life force that makes up the universe. I am one with my Father & I honor that same life energy in all that I meet.

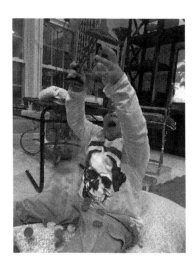

Why is play so important for adults?

It's because we can and should not be all work. Play creates a space for creativity. Fun provides vision.

Play relaxes the sub-conscious mind to allow new energy to get through all the serious and mundane thoughts that hold our creative process hostage.

Play relaxes the body and can even aide in healing.

Play makes you exhale.

Play brings you to a place of light & breezy. It puts a smile on your face. And guess what it improves all relationships.

So, go ahead. Put down your woes, purposes, agendas & plans for a moment to feel, see and attract something new.

Then go back to work...... (~_~)

Go For It: Play time is good for my soul.

WHO WE ARE NOW!

The soul needs success.

Who we are now is never an indication of who we can become.

We all have heard that circumstances do not define us.

Integrity and Accountability = Success!

Our brilliance, strength, talent and accomplishments are from God!

What will you do with yours?

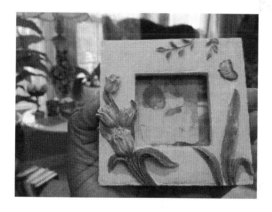

Go For It: Father may my gifts be a blessing to you and others as I am committed to becoming all that you have sowed into me.

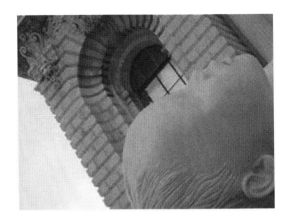

Are "**You**" missing from the whole plan....???

We sometimes feel that the people we see in the media are bigger than us and that they have a more glamorous life. We read their witty books, listen to their lectures and follow all their accomplishments on social media.

We act below our purpose because we do not realize the greatness our own lives can contribute to the Universe. Do you realize that each one of us is a part of the whole plan? This means that every small jester is so important because it snowballs into huge accomplishments for both you and others.

Please do not sell yourself short....

- ❖ **Your Smile**
- ❖ **Your Hello**
- ❖ **Your Gifts**
- ❖ **Your Life**
- ❖ **Your Purpose**

Go For It: I know and accept that my missing from the whole plan would be a tragedy for my little is much!

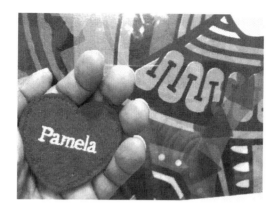

When is the perfect time to show someone that you love them?

I think every day is a perfect time to show that you care.

However, this love should not be directed to others only. You are the first person that should be loved by you!

You can give and receive the same from others when you make the health of your own heart a priority.

Are your thoughts loving for a healthy you? Are the relationships in your life harmonious for a healthy you? Are your boundaries clear for a healthy you?

Is your love......???

Healing

Energy

About

Loving

The

Harmonious

You

Go For It: I am worthy to receive a life time of the healthy love that I desire!

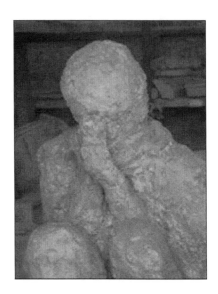

Why Pain and Possibility?

Pain and Possibility are two words that evoke emotions of dread or excitement.

Both words can bring you to tears.

Both words can create uneasy emotions.

Both words are powerful examples of your focus.

Both words are part of the human experience.

Both words can influence a similar outcome.

Pain can push you into Possibility.

Possibility can push you thru the Pain!

Go For It: Thank you Infinite Wisdom for helping me to push thru the pain into possibility.

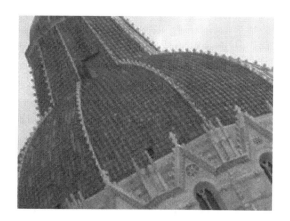

Mind Over Matter...... "Often hard to achieve"

Since we live in a physical world it is often best to get right to the matter, to help the mind shift the matter. Usually the matter is something that you can see, hear, feel or touch but don't know how to resolve. This is when doing something physical becomes so important.

Now the physical doesn't have to be about the matter either. The physical just needs to create movement. That energy or action causes a ripple effect for change when you move one thing. Therefore, I usually do something like wash my dishes. Or make the bed when I am stuck on mind over matter. When I am stuck on mind over situation, I need the meditative action of doing. This helps me to put the physical into submission to the mind so that an answer to the matter can be heard.

See matter or problems need to be distracted in the same way that a parent tricks a child into letting them remove a splinter or loose tooth. Now. Can you see the mind working in that matter?

Go For It: I turn every problem over to my Higher Source who is the real energy working on my matter for an achievable solution

The key is within

to create all possibilities!

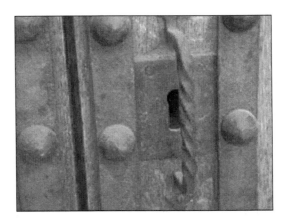

Go For It: I seek God's direction every day because that I the key to my success and accomplishments.

Today, I thought that I had nothing to write.

My thoughts are quiet, and fear is at bay.

I am feeling thankful and blessed.

I see all possibilities aligning.

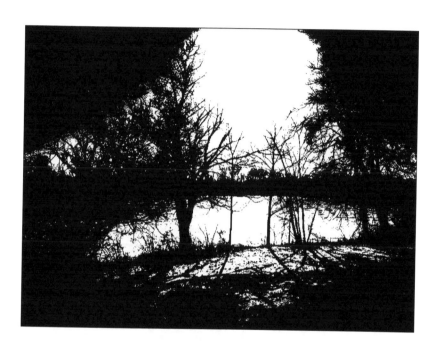

Go For It: I thank heaven above for thoughts that are in alignment with His goodness and merci regarding my purpose for today.

I don't think that God would do to us

what man does in the name of religion.

I choose to think that the Power

who created us in his own image

expects us to honor that part of him

in every person that we meet.

Wouldn't it be something

if that is the main reason

why we exist?

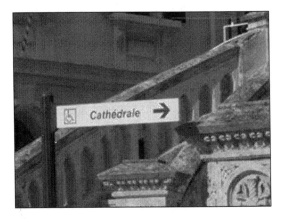

Go For It: Thank you Lord for the revelation that I alone am not more important than others and that my existence is connected in the way that we are all important to each other.

Peaceful is the time when all the earth is asleep & only those who wish to commune with Infinite Spirit are still awake.

We listen with ears that hear His voice in the silence.

We listen with feelings that hear His voice in their hearts.

We listen with eyes that see the manifestation of His love in our lives.

We listen with thoughts that see His mind.

We listen with expectation for instruction and correction.

Knowing that to think requires listening. And to listen doesn't require thinking.

To think is to listen.

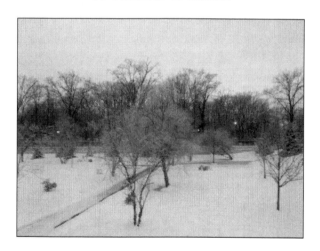

Go For It: I think to listen so that I can hear how much I am loved. I listen without thinking to hear how I am to love in return.

Those who have been in my home know that books are my Best Friends Forever (BFF) and are in "everyone" room.

This also includes "my" comic and coloring books. (~_~)

My nieces and nephews also have their own book shelf in my library. When they visit my living room floor becomes a play area for pillows, quilts, games, snacks and of course books.

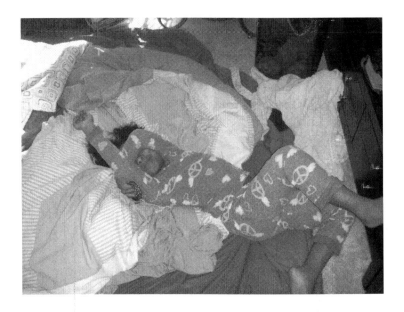

I think that the digital technological advancements are great. However, there is nothing like the weight of a book in my hand and the effect on my senses when I feel and hear the pages turn.

Or see the words, graphics and color take on a life of their own. What about the smell of a new book?

OMG, I'm drooling....!

For me this sensory experience connects me to the energy

of what I am reading in a very special way.

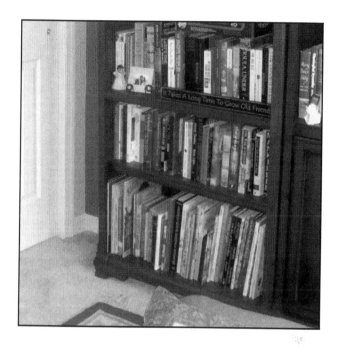

Go For It: Universe there are many spiritual books that provide in-site and instruction on how to live. Every day I will read something to drool over for a new revelation that will enhance my life so that I may be a blessing to others in my own way.

Focus on the outcome

and not the incoming distractions

that can derail your future success!

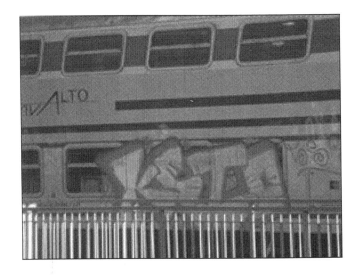

Real wealth is health from food infused with love during the preparation.

When you cook with mindfulness that energy transfers from you into the food to those who are eating. Although this may seem a little quirky, that energy becomes part of your blood which transfers vibrations thru the nutrients to your cells and organs. Today much more is known about the energy of the mind, body & spirit connection and how love heals.

Close your eyes and think about a favorite dish that your mom, dad, grandparents, friends, kids and others have made for you with intension. Doesn't that make you think "Lawd have merci", I miss Mama Jules's and Ma Smith's......!

Sorry I just drifted off because I feel the love. (~_~)

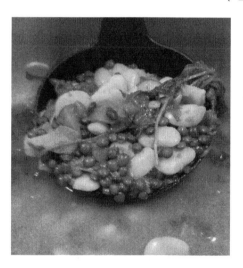

Go For It: I am mindful that my contribution to the universe can be a blessing when I choose to vibrate with love.

I am convinced that one of the reasons why we have a preoccupation with people, places and things outside of ourselves is because we are "Skin-Starved™". It's a term I use for needing love, affection and hugs in an appropriate way.

There is a growing population of single, married, widowed, young and aging people who are not being hugged regularly. The giving and receiving of touch is extremely healing for both adults and children. The exchange of energy in a hug can.

- ❖ Decrease anger and violence
- ❖ Lower depression and stress levels
- ❖ Improve the nervous system
- ❖ Boost the immune system
- ❖ Lower blood pressure
- ❖ Make you and others happy

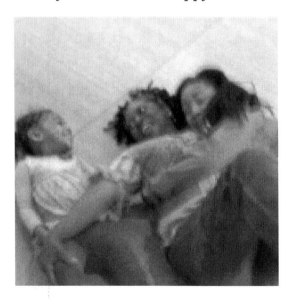

Go For It: Lord may my words, thoughts and actions give someone who needs a hug a little joy today.

Pee, Poop and Chew

Many of us who are animal lovers enjoy nurturing our four legged "Doys" and "Dirls", providing quality time, food and clothing.

But are we giving the same time, money and attention to a senior neighbor, mentoring a child or feeding a stranger? Are our pet relationships better than those with family, friends and strangers in need too? I know that pets are sometimes easier to deal with and love.

Yet, so are people with similar personalities. The difference is how we look at the experience. Animals chew, pee and poop on your favorite shoes, furniture and books.

People chew, pee and poop on your emotions, finances and time. However, with love, attention and some discipline to change behavior...they become bonding relationships for life.

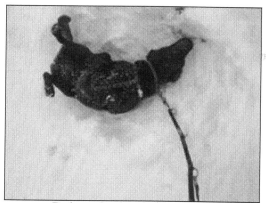

Daisy playing in the snow

Go For It: Father please help me to remember that pee, poop and chewing is a natural function of a healthy life.

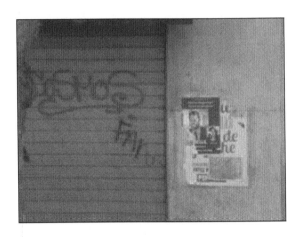

Signs and Wonders
"Photo 811"

Definition: "Cosmos - the universe seen as a well-ordered whole."

Please align me with the people, places and things that will help me complete the purpose we discussed before you formed us.

Have any of you noticed how specific words, songs, numbers and symbols appear repeatedly along your life's path?

You know the things that happen to provide comfort in a way that can't be explained.

For me the same words, scriptures, numbers and songs come up when I need guidance and confirmation that everything is in Devine Order.

This knowing gives me courage, strength and focus to keep moving towards my goals with encouragement and expectation.

Intuitively, there is a knowing that the people, places and things are aligning with the purpose that was discussed before I was born.

I took this photo on a whim several years ago when I was in Europe.

It is photo number 811.

Coincidences? Maybe!

However, ironically, it's the address of the house that my parents purchased when they moved us out of the projects hoping that this would provide us with better opportunities.

It is also the reoccurring number that appears in odd ways whenever I have a life change.

WOW!

Isn't it nice to know that something bigger than us has our backs! (~_~)

Go For It: Father it is comforting to know that you got me!

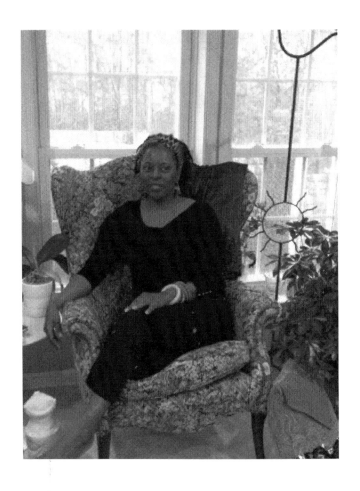

Recently I've been renewing my relationship with one of
my favorite items.

It is a wing chair that I found at a yard sale many years ago and purchased for $50.00. I upholstered the chair in a floral cotton tapestry that I found in a NYC shop that was going out of business for $5.00 a yard! I bought the entire "huge" roll.

What a find but you should have witnessed me bringing it home on the train!

This was during a time when I was working two jobs to pay the rent on my attic apartment until I had enough experience as an Interior Designer to earn a better income.

I would also stalk certain neighborhoods on junk day evenings...finding "free" stuff curbside which was loaded into my car, dragged home and "fixed up". I still call this trash to treasure design style "Early Attic™" and I have many of those finds to this day!

My wing chair is great for quiet reflection, reading, prayer and meditation. It is also a favorite place for visiting family and friends to sit while enjoying a glass of wine or cup of tea.

Gravitating to this area must have something to do with the fact that it is also flanked by other items from those that I love like the ceramic lamps from Mama Jules's bed room, Ma Smith's white marble vase from uncle Tommy's military service overseas and Jeffery Brown's wonderful candle stick holders which he used for many of his fabulous events.

I believe that spaces for moments when you need to calm the mind, body and spirit are so important for both adults and children. So, tell me...what area in your home soothes your soul?

Go For It: Lord, thank you for the creative peaceful space that is a result of my knowing you.

What connects us with the power

of the soul

for inside wisdom

to live in an outside world?

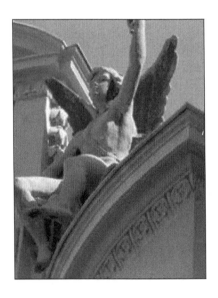

Your Inner Creates Your Outer!

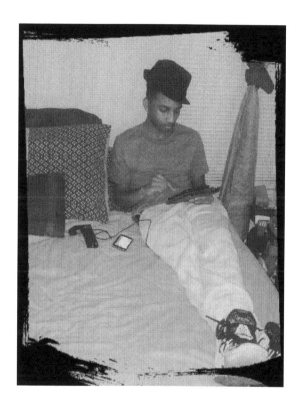

What are you feeding your mind, body and spirit?

Go For It: I am aware that I must feed my mind, body and spirit loving thoughts.

Too Much T.V. / "A Spiritual Distraction"

Too much T.V. is a spiritual distraction.

It deflects your attention away from what is important in your life.

 It gives you an outlet to become totally emerged in a false reality which keeps you from embracing your purpose.

It has become one of the little gods that separates you from relationship with God, self and others.

It blocks healthy thoughts and actions which could be an avenue to greatness.

Instead hours are lost on energy that which poisons the spirit and provides no productive outlet for success.

Moderation is necessary.

Censorship is necessary. Divorce is necessary.

Move the focus back to what is important.

The mind, body and spiritual service to self and others.

Go for It: Today I take a break from all distractions to focus on what is healthy for me.

Pray without ceasing to cease thinking that what God has for you is outside of His promise for your life.

Praying without ceasing is knowing that you are always connected to Source.

Know that we can talk and listen to God in both our awake and sleeping hours.

It is in our awareness that we can cease praying for things that are already ours. And take steps to be full of praise for what is already provided in abundance.

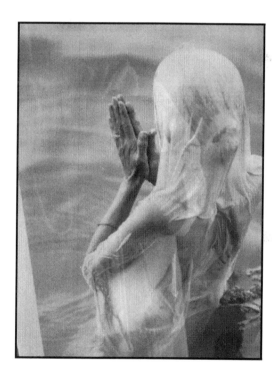

Go For It: I take comfort in knowing that all my concerns cease to exist because my Father provides a resource for every need.

Bumps on the Life Road / "Life's Twist and Turns"

Do you realize that there are many bumps and turns on the life road? Well I do!

It is not always easy to do the right thing at the right time when all the wrong people, places, things and emotions are tugging on or impacting your actions.

When this happens, it is so important to take a moment, a second, a pause and a breath to align your actions with the result that will produce the most good.

When you take a moment to pause and breathe – clarity and balance will override all the junk that may result in a negative outcome. Peace be still will allow you to find a space where you can organize your thoughts and feelings.

A pause for a second can keep you from speaking words that you can never take back. A single breath can provide fresh oxygen to the brain to help you write an appropriate response and then hit the send button. Or speak a gentler thought.

Navigating a rocky road or situation requires patience and skill. But it can be done successfully if you are determined and focused on getting to the other side, over the bridge (thoughts), threw the forest (emotions) with a heart for what or whoever will be the receiver.

Go For It: I navigate through life with consideration knowing that every day I meet myself in others along the way.

Soundness of mind and body should be a connection with our intuitive spirit.

Only I can create and perceive my own health.

Our health has a direct relationship with the Divine order of the universe.

Our thoughts set into motion a domino effect which impacts the whole universe, whether it be for good or bad, negative or positive, healthy or unhealthy.

Understanding a connection with our Creator and free will produces an energy which will set into motion a series of events that will impact the whole.

That is why consciousness is so important; all thought is relative. We are not independent of one another regardless of awareness.

Our responsibility for a motion that becomes an outcome happens even in our ignorance.

Go For It: Infinite Wisdom with your help may I be more aware that my emotional, spiritual and physical health impacts your plan for all of us.

The trials and challenges are present in my life to help my soul grow.

My soul or heart is like any other muscle that requires exercise.

My exercise here on earth in this vessel called a body is to face the challenges of my soul work. I know that working muscles is not always pleasurable. But the work is necessary to acquire the desired result.

So, from now on I will work with an expectancy for a good result. Even when I cannot see any progress, I will not become discouraged. I know that sometimes it takes many repetitions or tries through varied circuit training sessions to get a desired result. Oh, the pain of each exercise.

However, what joy on the other sided when the result is good. Therefore, I will focus on the result.

From now on I will trust my trainer, my God who is wiser than me. I will trust and believe that His instructions & coaching is always in my best interest.

When something is difficult I will talk to Him knowing that our hearts are one and He hears my thoughts.

Go For It: I (Your Name) am a beautiful creation of our most infinitely wise Father. He created me with everything that I need. I was born from His love. He holds me highly in His thoughts. Only good is petitioned from God to me.

Lack of obedience even as a free will choice always creates discomfort.

This discomfort leads you into a detour from your path.

It will challenge you to continue the search for your destiny.

Destiny hides in the core of each of us.

All destiny is an integral part of a collective life force.

My one thread influences the pull of another's heartstring.

It appears complicated.

But it is really very simple if you are quiet, so you can listen carefully.

There is always instruction in those quiet moments.

Go For It: Father, may I take time to listen and align my own purpose with yours to be a blessing to the collective energy committed to healing our world.

I do know that what I don't know; the Universe does.

This is when I need to rely on my faith. I am a mighty part of the Almighty Creator.

Therefore, I have the same unlimited intuitive ability because the Almighty Heart and I are one in consciousness.

This is my truth.

How I journey through life spiritually from a physical realm that has its matrix of limitations is my lesson.

I must learn to live in the moment focusing on faith, hope and grace.

This gives me the power and wisdom along with His love to accept this process as I journey towards my heart's desire.

Hear
Eternal
Answers
Realizing
Truth

Go For It: My faith keeps me focused on my Father as I journey towards my heart's desire.

Working out little challenges?

Good Morning!

Good Morning!

Life has a funny way of working out all challenges no matter how big or small.

Will you just relax into the flow allowing the principles of Devine direction to work out the details?

This Devine energy is all knowing and only wants what is good for us.

All we need to do is cooperate by walking in faith and not fear.... expecting good.

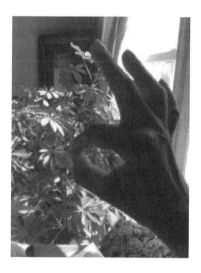

Go For It: What joy it is to know that my troubles already have a solution.

Let's focus on the true nature of God which is in all of us.

"LOVE"

"Beloved, let us love one another, for love is from God, and whoever loves has been born of God and knows God."
1st John 4:7

When there is balance in nature there is love. Love flourishes in many ways for healthy relationships.

Especially relationships with family, friends, strangers and self. Anyone who does not love does not know God, because God is love. Our relationships with one another will determine if our lives "S.H.I.P." no matter what is going on.

Showing
How
I'm at
Peace

A ship can glide through both choppy and still waters. This is how our relations should be with self and others.

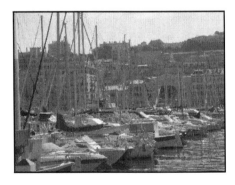

Go For It: Infinite Wisdom. My true peace is gliding through life's choppy waters loving my brother and sister as you love me.

Too Much!

"Is not necessarily enough"

✓ Can having everything be not having anything?
✓ Can seeing everything be seeing no-thing?
✓ Can loving too much be just as lonely?
✓ Can giving too much be a sign of poverty?
✓ Can eating too much be your starvation?
✓ Can working too much be a road to unemployed?
✓ Can having too much be not enough?

When we do anything to excess it becomes an unhealthy obsession...too much but not enough.

Too much but not enough happens when there is no balance in our lives for the whole man as in mind, body and spiritual needs. The mind, body and spirit know when there is excess and will work very hard to balance this problem.

That is why the very thing that you are obsessing over or having too much of will be the very thing to bring you to your knees if there is no harmony.

You can have too much of almost anything, but you must also pray, rest, eat, laugh, cry, hug, fellowship and love with balance.

I've found that all the things that we neglect when we focus on the too much are the very things that we need to be enough.

Enough is never too much.

Go For It: Today, I am in harmony with all the things that I love. I am in the new awareness that my balance of much is just enough.

When one loses a person to the final phase of life called death.

A barrage of questions regarding this natural phenomenon rises to surface in the minds of those who are left behind after that last breath.

How can something so natural cause so much fear and uncertainty?

We all want to know if there is an eternal passage of rites into the next dimension. Wouldn't it be comforting to know?

If the dead could speak we would ask them to elaborate on the process and clue us in regarding what we should do here to be accomplished over There. Whatever, that might be.

Scriptural text will give you many references to the There. But what is there? What if the There is exactly what you do here.

What if how one exits and how one lives their life here is parallel on some unseen dynamic dimensional plane there.

It is said that you can always tell the ending by the beginning.

Go For It: I commit to being a dynamic blessing here and only eternity knows of the best ending there.

Curtain Call! Last Call! / "The party is over!"

When is the party over for the things that you no longer want in your life? When is enough...enough? Are you tired of being sick and tired?

We tend to wait until things are so bad before we get the wake-up call to change whatever is keeping us from having the life that we want.

By birthright we are entitled to having the best life experience every day. The Universe only wants the best for us. But sometimes we do not see that for ourselves. Isn't it interesting that the Creator of man can want more for us than we the creations want for ourselves?

Please take some time today to sit down and think about one change that would give you the thing, chance, opportunity or desire you want in your life.

Once you identify one thing – write it down. Now ask for it!

Ask for the right people, places and things to help you achieve that thing.

It is yours!

You just need to ask and then believe it is so.

Go For It: Jehovah, I turn it all over to you for guidance to position me with access to the right people, places and things.

It is important to listen in the beginning of the day.

Before the mind starts to review all the worldly things that need to be done.

Before the world awakens us with all its survival energy, voices and thoughts.

Early morning is the time when nature and God commune to discuss the plan for man on that day.

They decide who will live or die.

What the weather will be like.

Which angels need to be in position to prevent an accident and so many more circumstances that pertain to all of Mankind?

The thing about listening and the importance is because while the angels, guides, nature & Spirit are talking...if you are still...you can hear the daily plan for your own life in the wind and in the silence of your thoughts while the earth is still.

Your connection to thought, will give you clear direction regarding your actions and will be grounded in peaceful productiveness for the day.

Go For It: I take time this morning to co-listen to the plans that the Universe has for my life today.

Presence is the Present

Now is the moment!

Your Presence is the present of the now moment.

Being in the moment creates a bond with

people, places and things.

It confirms that which is important in your life to help you

be the best present in the presence of another.

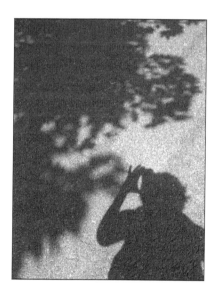

Go for It: Today I take a break from all distractions to focus on why it is important for me to be present to the presence of you and others.

Your soul path must be understood to orchestrate a harmonious coexistence with all life.

Beyond the layers or dimension of flesh, you will find cosmic congruity with yourself.

This understanding of self will reunite you with an internal dialogue with Spirit.

What you discuss is the key, for that is what will be propelled into motion throughout the universe.

The universal law only responds to what is put into motion by all thought.

Our responsibility is to safeguard our thoughts and to have a clear understanding of what is being projected by us for the best outcome.

There is good in all of creation because that was the original plan from the beginning. Some of us have forgotten our true self. Which is spirit.

Free will makes it possible for us to stretch emotionally, psychologically, socially, mentally, and spiritually by choice.

It is what we choose that brings us elevation.

Go For It: My inner conversations with self and spirit help me to be my best self every day.

The daily evolution of creative thought is power made available to us for soul work.

Soul work is an integral component of Creation.

Once understood, you will cease to struggle with the cyclical

journey for truth.

Life will be an adventurous expedition back to the Creator.

The physical expression of strife in this world will lessen.

However, do not deceive yourself. It will never go away.

It is the common denominator for all life.

It is to be used as a tool to measure your growth by the

choices made.

Go For It: I am a self-expressed co-creator of my life. I am thankful that I can take time to enjoy the adventure.

Choose your choices wisely for you will be held accountable.

Accountability comes in layers.

Those who are further along in the process will be reviewed

accordingly.

Intuitively you know who you are even if you do not answer

to the call.

What a Pity!

Because you will always feel the tug in your soul as you

maneuver through this life.

It is that tug which makes you uncomfortable in your temple

nudging you to choose your purpose.

Go For It: Father I choose to be held accountable for all areas of my life and take comfort in knowing that your tug guides me to my purpose.

Sin is a war raging between the consciousness of those

who see clearly.

And those who ignore this choice.

A sin conscious mind wants an easy fix.

Seeing
Into
Negativity

A clear mind works to manifest possibility.

Calm
Loving
Expression
Allows
Receiving

Go For It: I take responsibility for making great decisions with a clear mind.

Spirit can't pour into you when there are so many

conflicting thoughts going on in your head.

Silence creates a balance in the body to help you

receive with clarity.

Listen. Listen. Listen.

The answer to every solution is in your silence.

Use this gift to heal.

Go For It: Healing takes place in my life and issues are resolved when I am still enough to listen.

The "F" trap......

Fickle

Friends

Fathom

False

Frequent

Frequencies

For

Failing

Go For It: Father's favor funnels fortified fruit for fulfilling factual foreseen futures.

My house is your house is the spiritual mind of a soul worker.

Your temple is the vehicle by which your spirit can move, live and be. It is the structure that is vital for the soul's growth.

This includes both your physical temple on two legs (body) and the sanctuary (home/residence) both of which you live in.

Therefore, having a balance between the two is so important especially regarding what you put into each.

It is the place where you get to relax, rejuvenate and recharge.

Both require order, cleanliness, water, fresh air, light, peace and healthy nourishment.

What you put in each will impact your life.

Go For It: My house is filled with a life force that provides love, joy, peace, forbearance, kindness, goodness, faithfulness, gentleness and self-control.

Life has a way of tripping us up with surprises that can

throw us off our entire program or life path.

At least that is what we think.

However, this tripping is all part of the plan for your

purpose.

Confusion is a sign that the mind and spirit are balancing

options to help us move forward.

When there is confusion it is best to be still and to listen

intuitively to all possibilities before you act.

Go For It: I trust that my confusion will lift as I focus on your promise to be the guiding force in my life. I give up worry and fear for faith. It is then that I can work out all the details of my path according to your plan.

Most parents know intuitively that their children hear them even when they act like they are not listening.

So, it is with Spirit.

It will speak to you in that small still voice, planting that seed for you to listen to now or later.

It is not until you hear your own child repeat those exact words to the next generation or sibling that confirms they understand the concept.

So, it is with us.

When Spirit hears or see us practicing behaviors that are good for the collective whole – than it is clear the message seed has germinated & grown.

Sowed into a good open heart.

Sowing
Elevates
Every
Deed

Go For It: I willingly give my life over to serving with an open heart and mind.

God continues to show me that our agreement is being completed by Divine direction with help from the Universe.

People, places and things are lining up for my purpose.

I just need to stay focused and committed to my goals.

All things are possible if I just put one foot in front of the other and allow God to move in the right direction on my behalf.

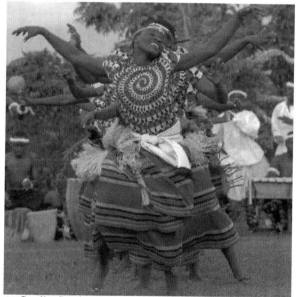
Photo Credit: Graduation - Set Her Free – http://setherfree.org

Go For It: I look forward with expectancy knowing that my steps are ordered and guided by a power greater than me.

The energy that we give to an expectation that satisfies the

ego instead of the Collective good will create confusion and

fall short of the goal.

What is the Goal?

Your Soul!

We are living in a time when each of us can contribute a

portion of our time, talent and gifts to

the world which are our communities.

Or to a person who is hurting.

When we function from the ego for praise and money we

ease God out.

We create a ripple effect even if no-one is watching.

Go For It: Infinite Wisdom I decrease my own words, thoughts and actions so that you may increase and magnify your vision by using me.

Why are we so hard on ourselves and others when we fall short if success and failure are the yin & yang opportunities for growth?

Wouldn't it be better to embrace the failure to determine what could be learned?

❖ Sometimes the best cookies are the burnt ones.

❖ The cake that fell apart makes a delicious parfait.

❖ The broken French fries taste the best.

❖ The book is a result of a failed relationship.

❖ The awful hair cut is now a new fashion trend

❖ The lay-off resulted in a new business

You cannot lose with failure if the lesson is learned because it is the very thing that will catapult you into success.

Go For It: I may not always like it, but I embrace failure as another chance to provide a foundation for knowing when something is finally right.

The Universal Collective mind of God with all its

Infinite possibilities will guide me to a blessing that

is more awesome than anything that I could

imagine for myself.

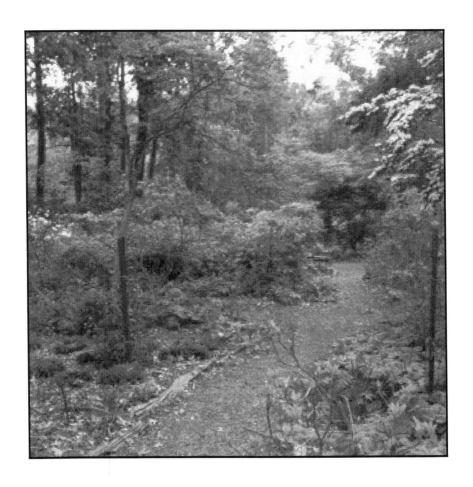

Sleep enticing little enchantress who holds the power of each new dawn in her hand.

She molds and shapes it according to her divine spell.

We are all powerless subjects in her hands.

We submit daily to abide in her truth as she leads us down new avenues of revelation and truth.

Who will seek her to know more about their self and own Divinity?

She holds you captive in a slow dance based on faith, releasing you with renewed strength each new day.

Follow her path. Take heed to her instruction.

Harken to the voice of a brand-new day; a new opportunity to stretch & grow. Thru her you can reach for the heavens to receive Fathers love.

A love so great that in His wisdom he created a way for you to prepare for greatness while you slumber. Sleep is his tool and a gift to all.

Who wants to receive true riches & glory while you rest?

Sleep is the creative prophetic metamorphous for dreams that come will true.

Go For It: In Sleep heaven sent wisdom flows down to me.

Do you know how it feels when a baby goes limp?

Especially when you hold it gently cradled in your arms

and

close to your own heart beat?

I Am That; the arms that hold you tight

I Am That; relax in me and give me your woes

I Am That; the spirit wind guiding you thru every obstacle,

problem and storm

I Am That; the same one who has your expected outcome

I Am That; your strength dear one who is close to my heart

So, retreat into my arms where there is peace.

My promises have already given you

everything that you

need!

Go For It: I hear you in spirit and harken to your voice. You are the I Am That I Am concerned about all your beloved sons and daughters.

Why is it that we can feel both excited & a wee bit jealous when we see someone finally achieving success?

Maybe it is because seeing their success reminds us of shortcomings regarding our own purpose.

I used to chastise myself when I felt that brief ping of why not me?

Until I realized that why not me was the universe trying to get my attention.

Why not me, was my responsibility to change my pity party to an achievement.

Although I genuinely supported another's dream. I also realized that I needed to focus & nurture my own for water to seek its own level.

Since I am in the company of rising water. This must mean that I can also float to the top.

The thing about floating is that you must do some work to get to the deep end.

And then relax and trust that the process causing you to float is adequate to guide you to your own success.

Go For It: I know that my success will seek its own level when I consistently put in the time and energy to stay focused on the goal.

LISTEN....

When the going gets tough you need to get up and keep going.

Now I know that sometimes this is hard to do.

However, one must continue to go on because it is important.

This will train your mind, body and spirit to never give up.

Your whole being will learn to roll with life's challenges.

You will get use to knowing that there is always an answer & solution to every experience.

Each experience will teach a different lesson. How you pass will determine your emotional, spiritual and physical growth.

You will learn that you are just passing thru on your way to the exit.

You will learn that the entrance and exit will have both joys and woes.

But isn't that simply life?

Go For It: I enter and exit all my situations with courage knowing that you can only pass thru something if you keep moving in faith.

Could it be that we are all from the same family of dough created with the same ingredients?

Think of a huge bowl of dough that makes many loaves of bread in different types of pans.

Some loaves rise and bake nicely, and others may not.

Sometimes situations like the correct oven temperature or opening the door frequently can impact the loaf.

We are all good dough in the eye of our Creator, even though situations, environment and other challenges can affect our lives.

I know for me that a slightly burnt lopsided loaf of bread can taste lovely with a smear of butter & honey!

Give someone you know a smear of encouragement to help them rise.

Deciding
Ongoing
Unconditional
Giving
Heals

Go For It: I offer myself in relationships to SMEAR love, kindness and encouragement towards those rising above all challenges.

101 Things...!

One morning I woke up with what felt like 101 things on my mind to accomplish.

However, Spirit said wait a second!

How about you allowing some time to be still and listen.

I had spent the weekend serving many others and I was very tired. But, I wanted to keep it moving to tackle the 101 things on my list.

Finally, I listened to that small still voice to rest after hitting the snooze button three times.

Unfortunately, for some of us work is rest and resting requires more work to achieve stillness.

However, it is when we rest that we can work on healing some things that working ignores like our mind, body & spirit.

Rest creates a space for creativity, restoration and healing.

Go For It: Sometimes the purpose of rest is to create a working space for healing things in our lives.

Greatness is a commitment to a vision that makes absolutely "no sense" to anyone else but you.

This "nonsense" is the reason why mountains have moved for people who did not look strong enough to pick up a full glass of water. Greatness is the willingness to accept that the very thing you desire is yours if only you believe.

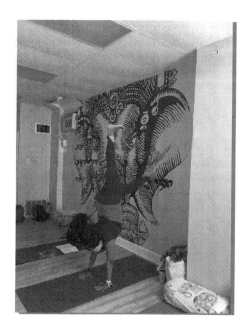

Go For It: Habitual consistency insures successful results!

The reason why some can see is because they still believe.

They believe in the impossible & things not seen by others.

It's a knowing that others cannot feel because you & the Creator can see possibility in manifesting the incredible.

For children this comes naturally until they are taught to doubt their own reality.

We have it all wrong.

Our kids come here to teach & help us grow.

We should watch, listen & respect them because they still have a direct connection to Source.

They also mirror & show us who we really are.

We think we are guiding, protecting and teaching them; but it is really us who will actually learn.

Go For It: Child of the Creator. What is real for you?

**It is in my vulnerability that I am open to share
all of me unconditionally.**

Vulnerability helps me to identify with others and it gives
them an open door to approach me to share, knowing that
there will be no judgement as we work thru similar shit!

When someone else has more to lose in a relationship the
other person may want to consider extending themselves
more to show commitment for feelings of inadequacy.

You should not be responsible for someone's happiness. But
sometimes kindness, support and love can heal by giving the
other person the strength to find out what God has already
provided to fulfill their purpose, vision and life goals

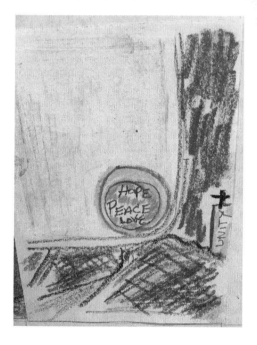

Go For It: In the beginning, middle and end I will try to
leave it better than I found it

Preparation to know thyself is an important vehicle for knowledge and productivity.

Serving also creates character and fulfils a purpose for the mind, spirit and body.

Why are we here? Could it be to recognize a common link between all lives?

Life is the most important energy and blessing from Infinite Wisdom. Understanding and respecting this will bring peace.

The ability to achieve is determined by our willingness to hear and submit. Submission is required to bring the body into stillness to understand purpose.

Common threads are linked from person to person. Each experience and incident are no accident but just a stepping stone to a higher calling.

Magnify the God in you and others. Reverence this love, peace and joy, by honoring the responsibility assigned to your soul.

The soul must always come first, or something is wrong.

Could this be why we come here in the first place?

My soul is grateful for any opportunity to stretch, give and grow closer to Him.

Go For It!

I hope you took what you needed!

Now go hug and play!

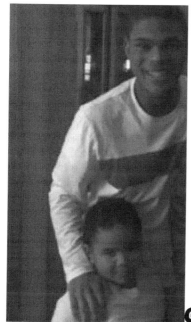

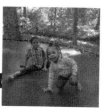

Go For It!

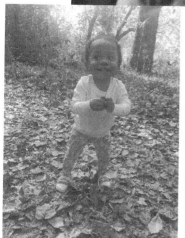

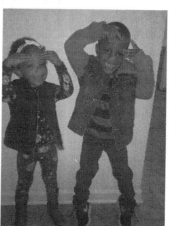

Hug & Play!

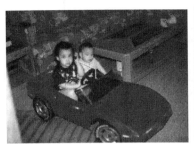
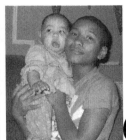

Go For It!

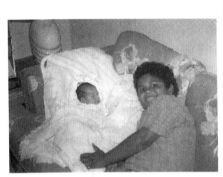
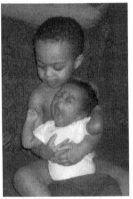

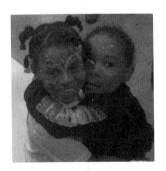

Hug & Play!

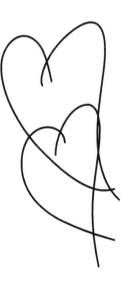

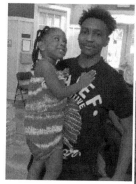

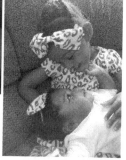

Hug & Play!

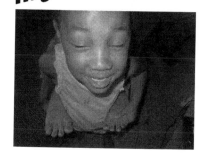

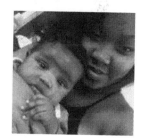

Go For It!

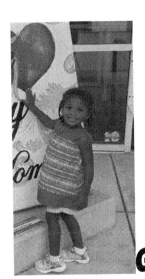

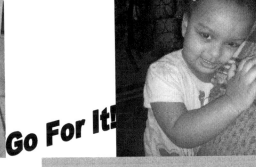

Go For It!

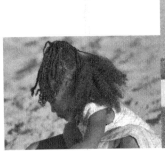

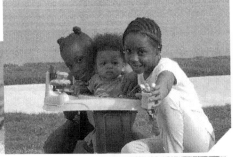

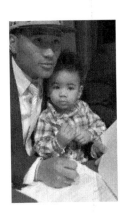

Hug & Play!

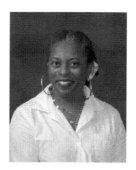

Pamela Rene' Slater has always had an interest in mind, body, spirit and living environment health & wellness.

She is a graduate of the Kean University of New Jersey BFA: Interior Design Program and has been working in the design community for over a decade.

Her experience also includes Integrative Nutrition Health Coach training from the Institute for Integrative Nutrition's (IIN) cutting-edge program. Studies included over 100 dietary theories, practical lifestyle management techniques, and innovative coaching methods with some of the world's top health and wellness experts.

However, she knows first-hand that organizing the living/work areas for total well-being in mind is so important! Her goal is to create spaces designed to balance the body, home and business for a good life & well-being by providing a co-creative approach utilizing both her interior design experience, yoga and integrative nutrition health coach training.

Workshops: "From Refrigerator Blues to Healthy Choices!", "Is Your Home Killing You?", "Your Inner Creates Your Outer!", "Gently Move It Yoga!" & "Simply Simple Interior Design Solutions!"

Wishing you a good life!